I0415544

The Smart & Easy Guide to Sleep Disorder & Insomnia Relief: The Restful Book of Therapies & Treatments for Sleeping Disorders, Insomnia, Narcolepsy, Restless Leg Syndrome, Night Sweats, Heartburn and Snoring in Men, Women and Children

Susan Jackson

Legal Stuff

COPYRIGHT

Copyright © 2013 Checkmate Marketing Group LLC. All rights reserved worldwide.

No part of this publication may be replicated, redistributed, or given away in any form without the prior written consent of the author and publisher.

Checkmate Marketing Group LLC

DISCLAIMER

THIS BOOK IS NOT DESIGNED TO, AND DOES NOT, PROVIDE MEDICAL ADVICE. ALL CONTENT ("CONTENT"), INCLUDING TEXT, GRAPHICS, IMAGES AND INFORMATION AVAILABLE IN OR THROUGH THIS BOOK ARE FOR GENERAL INFORMATIONAL PURPOSES ONLY.

THE CONTENT IS NOT INTENDED TO BE A SUBSTITUTE FOR PROFESSIONAL MEDICAL ADVICE, DIAGNOSIS OR TREATMENT. NEVER DISREGARD PROFESSIONAL MEDICAL ADVICE, OR DELAY IN SEEKING IT, BECAUSE OF SOMETHING YOU HAVE READ ON THIS BOOK. NEVER RELY ON INFORMATION ON THIS BOOK IN PLACE OF SEEKING PROFESSIONAL MEDICAL ADVICE.

THE AUTHOR, PUBLISHER AND ALL AFFILIATED PARTIES ARE NOT RESPONSIBLE OR LIABLE FOR ANY ADVICE, COURSE OF TREATMENT, DIAGNOSIS OR ANY OTHER INFORMATION, SERVICES OR PRODUCTS THAT YOU OBTAIN THROUGH THIS SITE. YOU ARE ENCOURAGED TO CONFER WITH YOUR DOCTOR WITH REGARD TO INFORMATION CONTAINED IN OR THROUGH THIS BOOK. AFTER READING THIS BOOK, YOU ARE ENCOURAGED TO REVIEW THE INFORMATION CAREFULLY WITH YOUR PROFESSIONAL HEALTHCARE PROVIDER.

LIMITATION OF LIABILITY

THE MATERIALS IN THIS BOOK ARE PROVIDED "AS IS" WITHOUT ANY EXPRESS OR IMPLIED WARRANTY OF ANY KIND INCLUDING WARRANTIES OF MERCHANTABILITY, NONINFRINGEMENT OF INTELLECTUAL PROPERTY, OR FITNESS FOR ANY PARTICULAR PURPOSE. IN NO EVENT SHALL OR ITS AGENTS OR OFFICERS BE LIABLE FOR ANY DAMAGES WHATSOEVER (INCLUDING, WITHOUT LIMITATION, DAMAGES FOR LOSS OF PROFITS, BUSINESS INTERRUPTION, LOSS OF INFORMATION, INJURY OR DEATH) ARISING OUT OF THE USE OF OR INABILITY TO USE THE MATERIALS, EVEN IF HAS BEEN ADVISED OF THE POSSIBILITY OF SUCH LOSS OR DAMAGES.

Table of Contents

Do I Have A Sleep Disorder? The Types, Signs & What You Should Know

Seven Warning Signs that You May Have a Sleep Disorder

The definition of a "sleep disorder" includes an extremely disrupted sleep pattern, with symptoms of: difficulty with sleep initiation (falling asleep), difficulty with remaining awake at appropriate times or falling asleep at the wrong times, excessive sleeping or other unusual sleep habits.

Determining whether or not you actually have a sleep disorder may require some professional help. But, read through these seven common signs of sleep disorders and find out if you may need to get more help.

1. Is it difficult for you to wake in the morning? Do you wake too early and find yourself unable to return to sleep?

2. Do you experience difficulty with concentration?

3. Do you fall asleep at work or while driving?

4. Do you experience feelings of depression, anxiety or excessive moodiness or irritability?

5. Do you experience unusual sensations in your legs during the night?

6. Does your family tell you that you have a snoring problem?

7. Do you wake frequently during the night?

If you have most or all of these signs or symptoms, then you may indeed have a sleep disorder. First and foremost, if you simply find that you are chronically exhausted and there is no other reason that you can think of (meaning you think you are getting enough sleep), then it is very likely that you have a sleep disorder. Feeling like you have been awake all night, or finding that you are awake all night, can be a huge problem when it comes to functioning throughout your day. It is well known that having poor sleep patterns can lead to major health problems.

There are four different stages for the sleep cycle. Hormones help to regulate the sleep cycles, and play a big part in keeping your metabolism regulated. When sleep disruptions chronically occur, the sleep cycle will be dysregulated and this is why you will feel so tired when you wake up in the morning, even after you think you have had a good night's sleep. One bad night of sleep will not cause you too much difficulty, but if you start to feel lethargic and exhausted, day after day, then it is wise to see your doctor to try and uncover some of the conditions that could be related to your issues, including a sleep disorder.

When concentration problems arise, or you notice that your reaction time has slowed, then you might actually be suffering from a sleep disorder. Because sleep is so critical to our overall health and well being, there are major problems that can arise from having too little. If you have a sleep disorder, it is very important that you get help from a qualified professional, so that you can continue to function! People who are chronically sleep deprived are not only at risk for health problems, but will be at a higher risk for car accidents, work issues, relationship problems and more.

Some people will have intermittent sleep problems that can be fairly easily attributed to a late night, using alcohol, having a stressful problem or some other explanation. This is not really a sleep disorder. It can become a sleep disorder when the problem becomes chronic, and the person begins to experience repeated sleep disturbances. As long as the simple problem (staying up too late, drinking alcohol, etc.) is handled promptly, then there is probably no reason to work. But, letting this problem get out of hand is when people get into real trouble and many aspects of their lives become affected.

Those who find that they are experiencing chronic moodiness and irritability, or even anxiety and depression symptoms, may be suffering from a sleep disorder. Although everyone experiences some degree of depression or anxiety on occasion, or feels moody and irritable, if there is not a known short-term reason for the emotional changes (stress, family situation, job situation, death of loved one, illness, etc.), then the issue should be examined more closely to make sure that a sleep disorder is not to blame.

Many people suffer from what is commonly known as "Restless Leg Syndrome." This is a condition which causes a person to feel a constant feeling of motion in their legs, often described as "creepy, crawly" or "pins and needles." Trying to fall asleep with this feeling can be very challenging, and it can even wake you up from a sound sleep, making restless leg syndrome a very real issue for sufferers, even though there is often no detectable physical cause.

Restless leg syndrome is not a terribly serious condition, but the fact that it can cause sleep problems or a sleep disorder makes it a big problem for those who suffer from it. It can also be a very big deal for the spouse or partner, as restless leg syndrome can be disruptive to those around the sufferer, too. In certain cases, medication may be helpful, so check with your doctor if you have restless leg syndrome affecting your sleep.

Snoring is something that most people simply consider to be annoying. But, they may fail to realize that it could often be a sign of something much more serious. Sleep apnea is often first suspected because of snoring. Sleep apnea is a very dangerous condition when left untreated, because the actual process involves a cessation of breathing while sleeping. If your spouse or partner reports that you seem to gasp for air while sleeping, or if you experience any type of choking sensation or wake frequently, you should consider seeing a doctor and being evaluated for sleep apnea. Several types of sleep apnea exist, including obstructive sleep apnea, central sleep apnea and also mixed type sleep apnea.

Frequent waking throughout the night is another significant symptom of a sleep disorder. Although there are certainly many reasons for waking up a lot during the night, including poor lifestyle choices (drinking, smoking, poor sleep schedule, lack of exercise, etc.), a sleep disorder may also be the reason. If you change your sleep hygiene and make improvements, yet you still find that you wake up many times during the night, then you may have a sleep disorder.

Women Suffer More Frequently From Sleep Disorders Than Men

It is estimated that nearly twice as many women as men experience sleep disorders. The sleep disorders that women experience affect their ability to fall asleep and stay asleep. There could be multiple reasons for this. Technically, a sleep disorder is an unusual sleep pattern that affects a person's functioning or health. Sleep disorders include problems falling asleep, frequent waking, inappropriate sleep times, excessive sleeping, or other sleep pattern abnormalities. Sleep disorders generally fall into four different categories: insomnia, disruptive sleep disorders, hypersomnia and dysregulated sleep patterns.

Women may be more affected than men for many different reasons. Because hormones play such an important role in sleep regulation, and women often experience more hormonal fluctuations than men, they are at a higher risk for developing sleep problems. Other things, such as stress, sleep conditions, pregnancy, menstruation, depression and anxiety may all play a role in sleep problems. Additionally, circumstances such as pain, worry or grief may also temporarily affect sleep, or even potentially have long term effects. Medication conditions may also play a role, as well as menopause or perimenopause.

One of the main issues with sleep disturbances related to menopause is the development of anxiety and heart palpitations. These are problems that can be triggered by low hormone levels. Symptoms that can occur include frequent waking during the night, night sweats or hot flashes at night, and insomnia. It is estimated that more than a third of women will experience these symptoms at the time of menopause—and often well before menopause truly sets in.

Pregnancy is a condition that only affects women, and it definitely affects sleep patterns. It is not a sleep disorder, but pregnant women can have sleep disorders. Many conditions can develop, including sleep apnea. Sleep apnea can be particularly dangerous for pregnant women, as the interruption in oxygen and the lowered oxygen saturation can adversely affect the fetus. Other problems that are commonly experienced by pregnant women include heartburn, backache, leg cramps, anxiety provoked nightmares, snoring and frequent urination. Each of these things will definitely have an effect on sleep patterns. Sleep is certainly very critical during pregnancy—women with sleep disorders are at a higher risk for low birthweight babies, preterm labor, preeclampsia and a host of other issues.

Older women are also highly likely to experience sleep problems. It is estimated that nearly 25% of women over 65 have sleep apnea. This condition is definitely more common in post-menopausal women. One contributing factor for sleep apnea is being overweight, and many post menopausal women struggle with weight issues, especially belly fat. This can cause sleep apnea, snoring and excessive fatigue.

Approximately one out of every five women report issues with restless leg syndrome. As discussed in the previous chapter, this condition can cause major sleep interruptions and lead to excessive fatigue, moodiness, irritability, anxiety and depression.

One very significant medical condition that can lead to sleep disorders is narcolepsy. Often first appearing during the teenage years, narcoleptic patients have abrupt sleep onset, often including a sudden lowering or loss of muscle tone. Nighttime sleep is often disrupted as well.

Generalized anxiety disorder is a condition in which chronic stress can be a contributing factor. This condition affects many more women than men, and usually results in significant difficulty falling asleep.

Nighttime pain can interrupt sleep. Nearly 25% of women report that they are awakened at least 3 times per week due to nighttime pain. Nighttime pain appears to be more common in women than in men and contributes to sleep disorders. Causes of pain may include migraines, other types of stress or tension headaches, pain associated with arthritis, or heartburn.

Insomnia is another form of sleep disorders that affects women more than men. Typically linked with depression and stress, insomnia affects many people. About one out of every five people with insomnia also suffer from major depression. Nearly all patients with depression suffer from insomnia and early morning waking that leads to further fatigue and exhaustion.

Because many women experience significant stress related to juggling many roles, such as mother, wife, caregiver, employee, etc., they are at a high risk for sleep problems related to stress.

Women who work different shifts are more likely to have difficulty getting enough sleep. Disrupted sleep patterns are more difficult to remedy when working shifts that do not follow traditional timing, such as the expected 9am to 5pm hours. Shift work adds strain to many family systems, leading to increased stress for women. When combined with physical factors, such as hormones, menstruation, and other female issues, this becomes significant. Pregnant women working different shifts may be at a higher risk for having low birthweight babies, having miscarriages or premature births due to the stress.

Nocturnal sleep disorders, such as those which cause someone to eat, sleepwalk or demonstrate other unusual behaviors while sleeping, are more likely to affect women than men. Most people with nocturnal sleep disorders have no recollection of their activities while sleeping.

Sleep Disorder Stats – Top Five Circumstances Caused by Lack of Sleep

Insomnia

Insomnia is a condition that results in significant difficulty falling or staying asleep. People with insomnia may not sleep for days on end. Insomnia is very common, and can last for one day, many days, or for a long time. The effects of insomnia are many, including fatigue, irritability, moodiness, depression and health problems. Lifestyle factors that may cause insomnia include drug and alcohol use, poor sleep hygiene, illness, stress, or even lack of exercise.

If you find that you are unable to fall asleep or stay asleep for more than a week or two, consult your doctor to evaluate whether or not you are suffering from a sleep disorder. Treatments are available that can help this condition.

Narcolepsy

Although rare, narcolepsy is a serious sleep disorder that requires treatment. The impacts of narcolepsy can be very severe, as falling asleep unexpectedly can be very dangerous. The most common symptom reported is excessive sleepiness during the day, combined with a nearly constant feeling of fatigue and exhaustion. Abrupt onset of sleep at inappropriate times is usually seen. Some with narcolepsy experience what is known as cataplexy, which is a sudden loss of muscle control that can lead to abrupt collapse. Injury can result from this condition.

Sleep paralysis occurs when a person is conscious but their body appears to suddenly "fall asleep." A person with sleep paralysis will be unable to move or speak, and may have hallucinations or dream-like periods with no physical control. The person may experience nightmares or be highly anxious that someone or something is prowling around them. This condition is very disturbing, as it can often be confused with many different serious mental health conditions.

Restless Leg Syndrome

Restless leg syndrome affects people in different ways, but it is generally described as a very uncomfortable sensation of movement or tingling in the legs. People with restless leg syndrome do not usually experience the situation unless they are sitting still or trying to sleep. Most commonly the sensation is felt in the calf area of the legs. Some relief may come from stretching or moving, but the relief is often only temporary. People with restless leg syndrome will usually have significant difficulty falling asleep, and it will also often interfere with the sleep patterns of the spouse or partner.

Other movement disorders, such as periodic limb movement disorder, can cause involuntary leg or arm movements while sleeping. Most people do not even realize that this is happening to them, although they tend to occur at regular intervals, such as every 30 seconds during certain phases of sleep. Even though the sufferer may be unaware, the movements may awaken them, leading to poor sleep and chronic feelings of fatigue, drowsiness and exhaustion.

It is important to rule out serious causes for involuntary movements, such as anemia, diabetes, arthritis or lung problems. Those with restless leg syndrome may find relief in massage or soaking in a hot bath before bed time.

Sleep Apnea

Sleep apnea is a serious medical problem that requires treatment. Left untreated, sleep apnea can result in death. Apnea causes the windpipe to collapse and obstruct breathing. Those with apnea typically experience significant problems with fatigue and drowsiness during the day. This leads to feelings of depression, often related to the fact that people with apnea demonstrate poor job performance. The lack of oxygen to the brain during the periods when the person stops breathing can lead to brain damage over time.

Apnea generally occurs as a result of over relaxation of throat muscles while sleeping. Treatments are available to prevent symptoms and even help reverse damage. Some of the things that are often recommended as treatment include weight loss, exercise, quitting smoking, oral and nasal appliances, and positive pressure machines. Surgical treatments may also be available in some instances for treatment of this dangerous sleep disorder, and symptoms should not be ignored.

Heartburn

Heartburn, or gastroesophageal reflux (GERD), results when the stomach does not properly digest food, and acid is forced back into the esophagus. Sufferers usually feel a burning sensation in their chest or the sensation of food coming back up with an acidic flavor. GERD can lead to asthmatic symptoms, coughing, hoarse voice or even symptoms that appear to be indicative of a heart attack. Heartburn may be increased while sleeping, and cause problems or a sleep disorder.

Sleep is Overrated - NOT! Why Us Mere Humans Need to Snooze

Sleep is an absolute necessity for the survival of human beings. It is actually possible to live for quite a while without food, yet not without sleep. All mammals, reptiles and birds require sleep to survive.

Scientists are not completely certain of all of the exact reasons for humans requiring sleep, but it is known that during sleep, most of the organs continue to function actively, as well as the body's regulatory systems. Certain parts of the brain are actually more active during sleep cycles. Hormones are produced during sleep.

Many scientists think that the brain is recharging during sleep. Because the brain changes function, and some parts will shut down activity during sleep, it may be a time for neurons to be repaired and synapses to rest and redevelop. After a long day of stress and thinking, sleep may be just what the brain needs in order to rest and reorganize.

During sleep, the brain can also actively perform tasks related to finding information and processing new information. Memory is reinforced with sleep, and learning is often solidified. Irrelevant and useless information may be purged during sleep as well. Because metabolism slows down during sleep, energy is conserved and may be redirected to the brain.

Our hearts and lungs also are permitted to rest during sleep. During sleep, blood pressure may be reduced up to 20-30% and heart rate may slow by 10-20%. This period of rest allows for the body to replace chemicals necessary for efficient function, and also repair muscle tissues and organ tissues or aging cells. The immune system can also be strengthened during sleep. Growth hormones are released while sleeping, which is especially important for children and young adults.

It is important that a body be well regulated on a circadian rhythm, and follow a 24-hour cycle in order to have the highest quality of sleep. During this 24-hour period, adults need approximately 7-8 hours of sleep for optimal functioning. This is the time that the brains glycogen resources are replenished, which is important for survival. Without the proper glycogen stores, the brain cannot function effectively during the day. This will affect memory, processing and overall regulation. Failure to follow a regular circadian rhythm can lead to inability to regulate body temperature, poor cognitive abilities, mood swings, hallucinations and more. Serious problems come from lack of sleep.

During wakeful times, the body drains itself of many of the chemicals required for functioning. Some chemicals vary widely during sleep, such as adenosine, which is required for efficient metabolism and preventing fatigue. Scientists theorize that sleep may be related to the evolution of the species and that the conservation of energy that comes with sleep is related to the "survival of the fittest." Primitive humans slept at night, developing this pattern, because it was easier to find food during the day and easier to take cover at night. Others think sleep may help the brain process information and experiences and develop memories.

Sleep is definitely a time for healing the body. During sleep, the body and mind has a chance to rejuvenate and restore itself. Long term memory is integrated during sleep, allowing memories to form and solidify.

In terms of evolution, humans are also sleeping and conserving energy at times when it would be difficult to find food. Sleep is regulated by hormones, such as melatonin, which increases during the evening hours in preparation for sleep. In the morning, melatonin levels are significantly lower. Another thing that helps to regulate sleep patterns and the circadian rhythm is light. Light waves help to reduce melatonin levels.

Problems with not having enough sleep include:

- Poor performance

- Poor concentration

- Poor reaction times

- Poor memory or memory lapses

- Increased risk of accident and injury

- Behavior problems

- Mood swings

Giving Pause to Sleep Paralysis – A Basic Overview of This Sleep Disorder

Those who are affected by sleep paralysis will be incapable of movement. They are unable to execute most voluntary movements once the onset of sleep occurs or just before waking. This is called either hypnogogic or hypnopompic. Those with sleep paralysis will be unable to move their arms, legs or trunk muscles. Often they will experience strong and vivid dreams, and even hallucinations in some cases. Many with sleep paralysis may report that they have the sensation of someone pressing on their chest, or the sensation that someone or something is prowling around them.

Fortunately, sleep paralysis episodes tends to be a short-term event most of the time. No lasting paralysis will occur and there are no specific risks to a person's health. However, the frightened feeling that are experienced, as well as the inability to move, can be very anxiety provoking and stressful, and the interruption of sleep can lead to other types of problems related to sleep disorders. Being uncertain of when the next episode will take place is also a very stress inducing factor.

Children tend to be more likely to experience sleep paralysis than adults, but there are plenty of healthy adults who will also experience sleep paralysis. Those who have narcolepsy or any other type of sleep disorder seem to be at a higher risk for sleep paralysis. Some speculate that sleep paralysis is a form of narcolepsy.

Narcolepsy causes people to experience uncontrolled sleeping, and often cataplexy as well. This is paralysis while fully conscious. Not all those with narcolepsy also have sleep paralysis, and not all those with sleep paralysis have narcolepsy, but they do often go hand in hand.

What Happens During a Sleep Paralysis Episode?

Scientists who have studied those who suffer from sleep paralysis use polysomnography to evaluate the body during the episodes. During sleep paralysis, the body will often demonstrate a sudden and dramatic lack of muscle tone. The sleep stage of REM is quickly achieved and the person experiencing the episode shows a dissociated and disregulated sleep pattern.

If you suspect that you are experiencing episodes of sleep paralysis, you should slowly attempt to move your extremities, and attempt "smaller" movements, such as blinking of the eyes or looking around. Many report that their movement freely returns upon waking or regaining consciousness. This may occur when a person is touched or hears a loud sound. Moving your fingers may also help to restore wakefulness and end the sleep paralysis episode.

If gentle movements are not helpful for restoring freedom of movement, you may want to try using the "shout and roll" technique. This may offer some people considerable success at stopping sleep paralysis episodes. To use this method, vocalize loudly while you roll your shoulders actively. This can help a person regain muscle control and full consciousness.

Experiencing sleep paralysis can lead one to have significant anxiety about sleep, and this can interfere with their ability to have a truly restful sleep. There are no known cures for sleep paralysis, but it can often be minimized by making sure that you consistently get enough sleep, practicing a healthy lifestyle that includes plenty of exercise and avoiding drugs and alcohol. Keeping stress to a minimum can also help to prevent sleep paralysis.

Some who experience sleep paralysis report that adjusting their sleep position can help to prevent episodes, or at least reduce the frequency. Most who experience sleep paralysis report increased episodes while sleeping on their back, yet fewer episodes while sleeping on their sides with proper support. Experiment with different positions to find which positions help you to have fewer sleep paralysis episodes.

Those who experience at least one episode of sleep paralysis per week, lasting over a period of six months or more, are described as having a "severe" condition. These severe cases may be treated with certain medications, such as antidepressants. For those who have sleep paralysis that is suspected to be related to cataplexy or narcolepsy, SSRIs may be helpful.

Causes of Insomnia in Senior Citizens

Those who have difficulty sleeping on a regular basis are said to have insomnia. This is probably the most common sleep disorder that is reported. Those suffering from insomnia report frequent waking, difficulty falling asleep, and waking too early in the morning. This condition is difficult for those who experience it, as there often seems to be no "good" reason for the sleep problem. When left untreated, chronic insomnia can lead to major health problems, as a chronic lack of sleep is very unhealthy.

Insomnia can affect both women and men, and people of all ages. It does tend to occur more often in women than men, and more often in senior citizens than young adults. Nearly a third of all senior citizens report insomnia, and two thirds of people over the age of 50 report having some type of sleep disorder. Senior citizens require between 6-½ and 7-½ hours of sleep per night for optimal functioning throughout the day.

When a person experiences long term, chronic insomnia, the body and the brain do not get the amount of rest that is necessary for proper functioning. A person is also at a very high risk for health problems. Short term insomnia is experienced by most people, at some point in their lives, often as a result to a situational stressor such as job stress, relationship problems, divorce, death of a loved one, or even positive stressors such as vacations or weddings. This type of insomnia is not terribly concerning, and will often pass after the situation changes.

Insomnia in senior citizens can have many causes. Things that affect sleep for senior citizens include stress, anxiety, illness, depression, drugs and alcohol, caffeine use, smoking, physical illness, arthritis, daytime naps, poor sleep hygiene, boredom or lethargy. Stressors such as anxiety, depression and grief can cause insomnia for seniors. Physical problems, such as painful arthritis, respiratory issues, diabetes, kidney problems, hypoglycemia, or hypothyroidism can all contribute to the insomnia of senior citizens. Restless leg syndrome may also contribute to sleep disorders. While everyone experiences the occasional night of "tossing and turning," when it becomes a chronic issue, then it should be fully explored so that any serious healthy or emotional problems can be ruled out.

For seniors, depression can be a major contributor to insomnia. However, it may not only keep a person awake, but it can also cause a person to sleep for too long, as a way of avoiding dealing with problems. Lifestyle choices, such as poor nutrition, alcohol use, caffeine and poor exercise habits can all contribute. Alcohol, especially, can be a problem since it is actually a depressant drug that can seriously interfere with sleep patterns. Also, the stimulant effects of nicotine and caffeine will interfere with healthy sleep. Each of these things can interrupt normal, healthy sleep patterns and cause insomnia.

Poor exercise habits can be a major contributor to insomnia. For those who experience insomnia with no known reason, one of the first recommendations is to increase exercise levels, with regular activity during each day. It has been scientifically proven that moderate levels of exercise, such as a 30 minute walk three or four times per week, can significantly improve sleep and reduce insomnia. More than half of the people who suffer from insomnia are likely to be helped by improving their exercise habits.

Seniors may have insomnia due to other issues, such as being overweight, having painful conditions such as arthritis, or having problems with mobility (difficulty getting around effectively).

Although insomnia is not a disease, it is a serious problem for those who suffer from it. It may also be a symptom of something far more serious, and if insomnia persists, it is critical that you see your doctor to rule out any major health conditions or underlying physical reasons that would explain why you are having trouble sleeping. If lifestyle changes do not positively affect the condition, then have an evaluation by a medical professional.

Restless Leg Syndrome and Sleep Disorders: What to Do About It

When it comes to sleep disorders, restless leg syndrome is a serious problem. This condition will cause sufferers to feel movements and tingling in their limbs, particularly their legs. The sensation may also occur in the trunk area. Some report throbbing and/or stinging, as well as the "creepy, crawly" sensation.

Individuals with restless leg syndrome tend to report an increase in their symptoms when they are less active, making specialists believe that increasing activity can improve the symptoms of those with restless leg syndrome. Avoiding long periods of sitting or standing still can help improve the situation. In most cases, the symptoms only appear while sitting still, and mainly at night while lying in bed, which is why it is often addressed as a sleep disorder. One or both legs may be affected by the problem.

Restless leg syndrome primarily occurs at the beginning of a sleep cycle, or in the early morning hours just before waking. When this happens, individuals with restless leg syndrome will often wake too early, and feel drowsy and exhausted all day long. Those with restless leg syndrome usually feel that they must constantly move their legs to try and alleviate the crawling and tingling that they feel, which severely interferes with healthy sleep patterns. It can also be a painful problem, in addition to being just uncomfortable.

Having restless leg syndrome is a common cause of insomnia. The irritation and distraction of the tingling and crawling sensation will often prevent a person from being able to fall asleep or prevent them from being able to stay asleep for a sustained period of time. This can ultimately result in a serious sleep disorder, and will lead to major problems—not limited to drowsiness and/or fatigue during the day.

Nobody truly knows exactly what it is that causes restless leg syndrome, and the true roots of the problem are unknown. There are some patterns that have been identified, however. Those individuals who have low iron levels or anemic conditions are at a higher risk for having restless leg syndrome. This means that women are at a higher risk than men, generally speaking, because these problems are more prevalent in the female population. Restless leg syndrome also tends to run in families, so if there are others in your family who suffer from this condition, you may be at a higher risk for developing the problem. Those who are overweight, or who have certain health conditions, such as diabetes or arthritis, are also at a higher risk for restless leg syndrome. Smoking, as well as heavy caffeine intake can also increase the risk.

Some serious health problems are associated with restless leg syndrome. It is important to be evaluated by a medical professional if you are demonstrating symptoms of restless leg syndrome, because, although it may only be an annoying problem, it could be indicative of a more serious underlying cause. Some of the associated problems include hormonal problems, kidney disease, nerve problems, and polyneuropathy. There are many prescription medications that are associated with restless leg syndrome, such as antidepressants, Zantac and Tagamet.

Restless leg syndrome can affect people of all ages, though it is often older adults who are more significantly affected. In children, restless leg syndrome is often described as something akin to growing pains. Restless leg syndrome in children may also be misdiagnosed as hyperactivity.

Similar to restless leg syndrome, periodic limb movement disorder in sleep also involves involuntary movements of limbs while sleeping. Arms and legs may bend in regular intervals, with jerky movements every 20-30 seconds. Like restless leg syndrome, this can cause serious interruption of sleep and lead to other kinds of health concerns once sleep deprivation sets in.

With no specific cure, restless leg syndrome is extremely difficult to effectively treat. Determining whether or not there are any serious underlying causes is very important. Blood tests and even x-rays may be ordered to rule out any specific reason for the problem. Determining whether iron levels are adequate or not will also be critical and can be determined through blood tests.

Smoking, drinking and consuming caffeine products will all increase restless leg syndrome symptoms. These are lifestyle choices that can usually be changed with some effort on your part. Adding in improved sleep hygiene habits and adding in routine exercise and activity can all help to improve the symptoms of restless leg syndrome and keep it under control to avoid having sleep disrupted.

There are some medications that are thought to be helpful for serious cases of restless leg syndrome. Medications such as ropinirole, gabapentin and tramdol may help. Other non-medication treatments may include acupuncture, chiropractic treatments, electric nerve stimulation and even adding magnesium supplements to the diet.

Narcolepsy: Causes, Treatments and Cures of This Sleep Disorder

Although it is one of the more rare sleep disorders, narcolepsy gets a great deal of attention because it is a very serious disorder. The risk of a person falling asleep unexpectedly at any time is very serious. This is a true medical condition. Falling, dropping what you are holding on to, or becoming limp suddenly is dangerous. This is a traditional neurological disorder that is thought to be caused by a disturbance in normal sleep-wake cycles and the brain's ability to adjust to these disturbances.

There are three very distinct symptoms in the condition of narcolepsy. One is known as cataplexy, which refers to the muscle weakness and paralysis that occurs suddenly. The person remains conscious when this happens. Another symptom, hallucinations that are experienced either while awake or right at the time a person is falling asleep, is referred to as hypnogogic and hypnopompic hallucinations. The third symptom that is indicative of narcolepsy is sleep paralysis.

Narcolepsy can cause very severe problems and affect the quality of life. People with narcolepsy typically feel very exhausted during the day and feeling very irritable.

Those with narcolepsy may experience multiple attacks per day, and these attacks can last from only a few seconds of nodding off to a long, hard sleep that can last up to an hour. A person with narcolepsy is at a higher risk when sitting down and relaxed, so long lectures or even driving can be a problem for these patients. After a narcoleptic episode, a person usually reports feeling refreshed. Those with narcolepsy may also feel like the attacks are somewhat hallucinogenic.

Narcolepsy affects approximately 25 out of every 100,000 people. There are nearly 150,000 people in the United States alone that have been diagnosed with narcolepsy. Scientists think that some people may be predisposed to the condition, as it is known to run in families. Narcolepsy typically develops during adolescence, and will often become obvious during the teenage years, between the ages of 10 and 20. In more rare instances, a person could be diagnosed with narcolepsy in childhood. Also rare, senior citizens could develop narcolepsy and have sudden onset of sleep as well. It is thought by most medical professionals that narcolepsy can become less serious as a person ages, but this is unproven.

To diagnose narcolepsy, a person's symptoms are reviewed by a medical professional. Typically an electroencephalogram (EEG) is performed, to measure the brain activity and rule out a seizure disorder. The examination is conducted in a sleep lab. Narcolepsy has no cure, but there are treatments that generally involve making lifestyle changes, including increasing exercise, avoiding drugs and alcohol—particularly stimulant drugs, and taking naps on a regular basis to help prevent the sudden sleep attacks.

Napping has been shown to help control the sudden onset of sleep attacks. Those who take 2 or 3 short naps per day may be less drowsy during the day, and better able to control narcolepsy. Some sufferers have been able to explain the medical condition to their employers and work this napping schedule into their day, to increase productivity and safety.

Daily exercise is also known to help with narcoleptic symptoms. Studies have shown that as little as 20 minutes per day of exercise can help to control the sleep attacks and improve the overall quality of a person's sleep. Exercise will also help with weight control, and, since those with narcolepsy who are overweight may suffer the most, this is certainly something that can help. Exercise should be avoided just prior to bed, along with alcohol, drugs, and smoking, to ensure that the body is fully able to rest comfortably.

There are several medications that are known to help sufferers of narcolepsy. Stimulants, including ephedrine or amphetamines may help with staying awake during the day. Antidepressants may be helpful, and can help with associated problems, such as the cataplexy experienced during daytime sleep attacks in narcolepsy. Most over the counter medications are not known to be helpful for handling the significant difficulties associated with narcolepsy. A newer drug, Modafinil, was approved in 1999 to treat the daytime drowsiness in narcolepsy. While it has been shown to be helpful for the daytime drowsiness, it does not usually show effectiveness for the other symptoms, such as cataplexy or hallucinations.

Narcolepsy is not a deadly condition, except for the fact that a sudden onset sleep attack can be very dangerous and lead to falls, accidents or serious injuries. Narcolepsy will usually cause significant interference with the person's ability to complete everyday tasks. Additionally, those who suffer from narcolepsy may be at risk for certain health conditions, including high blood pressure, depression, or other issues. Every effort should be made to maintain healthy sleep patterns, which will help to decrease the problems associated with narcolepsy.

Are You Having Problems Related to Sleepwalking—What You Should Know

Sleepwalking is an unusual problem, because it can be very unsettling to go to sleep in one place and then wake up somewhere completely different. Some sleepwalkers will go to sleep and wake up in their own bed, however, only to find out from their family members that they have had plenty of adventures during the hours in between. Sleepwalkers have no recollection of the events that take place during their sleepwalking.

Although this does sound incredibly strange, it is not uncommon. Approximately one out of every 10 people has experienced sleepwalking, some on a regular basis. The incidence seems more common in children. The medical term for sleepwalking is known as somnambulism. You have probably heard that you should never wake someone while they are sleepwalking, but this is not true. Sleepwalking itself is not dangerous, but those who are walking around while they are not conscious are at a high risk of injury, or of hurting someone around them.

When someone is sleepwalking, they appear to be awake and totally conscious. It can be difficult to detect the symptoms of sleepwalking. To determine whether someone in your family is sleepwalking, try to look them directly in the eye. If they seem to be staring back blankly at you, they may be sleepwalking. If they do not watch your movements and move their eyes, then they may be sleepwalking. Unusual behaviors or speech patterns may be present.

Many sleepwalkers will talk or mumble incoherently while sleepwalking. Most sleepwalkers are confused if they are awakened. Some may act aggressively toward the person waking them up, which is where the idea that it could be dangerous to wake a sleepwalker comes from. You should always wake a sleepwalker if they seem to be making an attempt to go outdoors or begin an activity that could cause injury (preparing food, using tools, etc.).

One of the biggest contributing factors for sleepwalking is a severe lack of sleep. Sleep deprivation can lead to many unusual behaviors, including sleepwalking. Lack of sleep will cause a person's overall level of consciousness to be affected. Those who experience severe fatigue are also at a higher risk. Additional issues, such as major stress, anxiety, depression, grief and other problems can also increase the likelihood of sleepwalking.

Sleepwalking can also be caused by certain medications, alcohol use, drug use or certain health conditions that are known to interfere with healthy sleep patterns. Children with asthma are at a higher risk for sleepwalking episodes because asthma is known to interfere with healthy sleep patterns. Those with sleep apnea are also at a higher risk.

The diagnosis of sleepwalking is pretty straightforward, particularly if the person has been seen sleepwalking. It is usually the family that is able to provide the most information about the sleepwalking episodes, as they are the ones who have seen the sleepwalker in action and can recount the stories. For those who live alone, sleepwalking can be a more mysterious diagnosis to make until you have gathered enough evidence to prove that there have been some nighttime adventures.

Determining the cause for sleepwalking is important for planning the treatment. The first recommendation is usually to get more sleep, on a more regular pattern. It is also important that, if you suspect sleepwalking, you try to make the environment as safe as possible by removing obstacles or locking doors to help minimize injury. Taking more significant measures, such as removing the knobs from the stovetop, or storing sharp objects carefully may also help to prevent further problems and keep the sleepwalker from harm.

Sleepwalking can lead to increased daytime drowsiness and fatigue, because it will definitely affect a person's ability to have a good night's sleep and be rested. Some may require sleeping medication or tranquilizers to help prevent the problem from occurring. Hypnosis has been shown to work for many patients. A combination of hypnosis and medication can be very effective for treating chronic sleepwalking, once serious health conditions have been ruled out.

Good sleep hygiene requires a regular routine, particularly surrounding bedtime. Being able to relax and fall asleep at the same time each night, and waking at the same time each day, is ideal. Try a warm bath at night, reading a relaxing story and avoiding any alcohol or stimulants toward the end of the day. A good bedtime routine can make all the difference in the world.

Because sleepwalking is usually caused by not getting enough sleep, developing those good bedtime habits may be all it takes to remedy the situation. Sleepwalking, by itself, is not seen as a dangerous condition and it is usually fairly easy to take care of. If sleepwalking continues to be a problem, you should seek medical attention before it becomes too serious.

Snoring and Sleep Disorders—A Problem For Many

Many people think of snoring as a funny problem, an unusual sound that someone makes while sleeping. Jokes about snoring are endless. But, the reality is, that snoring can be a symptom of a serious problem and should be checked out. There are many underlying conditions with snoring as a symptom, so it is important to rule these out before considering snoring nothing more than an annoying nuisance. Those who snore are likely to be having some type of sleep difficulty, and probably not getting the rest that they need. Snoring also is not only a problem for the person who is snoring, but it will cause serious sleep interruption for a spouse or bed partner, and possibly even other people in the house, if serious enough.

Different Levels of Snoring

Those who experience mild snoring may have nothing more serious than a congested nose, making their breathing much louder during sleep. Other snoring may be caused by certain obstructions, such as large tonsils or adenoids. Snoring may also be caused by the overuse of alcohol, drugs or certain sedatives. Most cases of snoring will fall into the "mild" category, and often a simple lifestyle change, or even a change in sleeping position to a side position, can help tremendously. Many cases of mild snoring are transient in nature, and related to a cold, allergies or temporary sinus condition. If this is the case, the snoring should improve once the other symptoms pass.

For those who experience more severe snoring, the possibility of having underlying health problems significantly increases. Those who snore regardless of their sleeping position, those who wake themselves with snoring, and those who are having very fitful sleep as a result of snoring, should consult their doctor to try and determine if there is a physical cause for the snoring.

Severe snoring may actually be sleep apnea, not just regular snoring. The sounds that a person with apnea will make while gasping for air during sleeping are similar to those that a person makes while snoring. However, those who experience snoring only (without apnea) are not pausing their breathing. Those with apnea may pause breathing for up to 10 seconds, which can lead to very dangerous and chronic health problems.

Some apnea sufferers will have up to 30 episodes during the course of one night. This amount of oxygen deprivation will have a cumulative effect. Not only will the person awaken frequently and have seriously disrupted sleep, but they will be losing oxygen, critical to the brain and organ function. Many with sleep apnea are not aware of the problem until it is pointed out to them by a spouse or partner. Sleep apnea can lead to fatal health problems, if left untreated.

Social Problems Related to Snoring

Although this may sound minor, snoring can be a social problem as well as a sleep disorder or medical problem. A snoring person will interfere with the sleep of their spouse or partner, and having another person's sleep interrupted will only make the problem worse, and potentially lead to health problems for that partner. The partner may not only worry about the person snoring, but may suffer symptoms of sleep deprivation themselves, leading to irritability, depression, fatigue and other problems that can affect the relationship considerably over the long haul.

Health Problems Related to Snoring

Chronic snoring can be a symptom of very serious medical problems. Sleep deprivation is known to be related to many health conditions, including obesity, diabetes, high blood pressure, heart problems, and possibly even stroke.

Some who snore are unaware, if they do not wake themselves up enough or do not share a bed with a partner. The effects of snoring include significant daytime fatigue, drowsiness, poor energy levels, lack of concentration and a weakened immune system. This makes a person far more likely to become ill if exposed to germs.

Snoring also means that the full oxygen available is not getting to the brain and the organs. This can lead to slowly developing brain damage, high blood pressure and more.

How Can You Reduce Snoring?

Lifestyle changes are the first suggestion for treatment of snoring, in most cases. Avoiding smoking, alcohol and drugs are obvious first steps toward improving any health problem. Some suggest that dairy products should be limited, as well, as they are often though to lead to increased congestion for some people. Weight loss and exercise are also thought to help reduce snoring for many people suffering from this condition. A change in sleep position, to a side sleeping position, is often helpful for reducing snoring. For those who move about frequently while sleeping, using supportive body pillows can help to maintain the proper position. A flatter pillow that helps to open the airway is also helpful for many.

Night Sweats and What to Do About Them

Medically known as hyperhydrosis, night sweats can lead to major sleep disruptions and cause the same symptoms as many other sleep disorders. Those who wake in the middle of the night, covered in sweat or feeling clammy, are experiencing more than just an annoying nuisance. Some with night sweats actually have to get out of bed, change their clothing and change their sheets before returning to bed. This can, obviously, be very disruptive to a good night's sleep.

Determining whether or not you are having night sweats is fairly simple, as it will be pretty obvious by your wet clothing and sheets. Night sweats alone are not always a cause for concern, and many people will experience them at some point during their lives. However, a person who is experiencing chronic night time sweating may have an underlying health problem that should be checked out thoroughly by their doctor.

There are many causes of night sweats. One of the most common causes of night sweats is menopause in women. The hormonal fluctuations that occur can affect body temperature, and cause night sweats or hot flashes while sleeping. Night sweats, however, are certainly not limited to women, as men can experience them, too. Although men do not go through menopause like women do, they will still experience hormonal fluctuations as they age and may have accompanying night sweats as a result.

Many sleep disorders are associated with night sweats. Sleep apnea is known to occasionally cause night sweats. When a person stops breathing while sleeping, they may begin to sweat as a result. For those who experience numerous episodes of apnea during the night, the resulting amount of sweat produced can be significant.

Any disruption in sleep can cause sweating as a result. If you are finding that you frequently wake during the night and feel sweaty and clammy, sleep apnea may be to blame and you should definitely contact your doctor to find out if that is the case. Treatments are available for this condition, and it should not be left untreated.

Many chronic and serious health conditions are known to cause night sweats. Any type of illness that has fever and chills as associated symptoms may be to blame. Many conditions that weaken the immune system, including HIV, AIDS, tuberculosis or Hodgkin's lymphoma can cause night sweats. Those who are receiving chemotherapy may experience significant night sweats, along with serious insomnia. Any condition that changes the overall body chemistry can lead to this problem.

There are many medications that can contribute to the presence of night sweats. Certainly any hormone medications, or hormone replacement medications, including birth control pills, can lead to night sweats.

Chronic health conditions, including diabetes, hyperthyroidism, anemia, seizure disorders, migraines, cerebral palsy or head injury can cause a person to experience night sweats, as well as any health problem that can cause a fever, such as infection.

Because night sweats can be caused by a myriad of health conditions, it is important that you consult your doctor if you experience night sweats on a regular basis. A complete physical may rule out underlying serious health concerns and help the doctor to determine the best course of treatment for this condition.

Primary hyperhydrosis is a rare condition but will cause very heavy sweating, both during the day and at night. This is a condition that can interfere with many aspects of a person's life. Treatments are available, including surgery to remove some sweat glands and limit the amount of sweat that is produced.

As with all other sleep disorders, there are lifestyle changes that you can try to limit the amount of night sweats that you are experiencing. Obviously, the first step is to establish good sleep hygiene habits and get regular sleep and rest. Also, avoiding alcohol, drugs and smoking can help.

Some think that there may be an association between eating spicy foods and experiencing night sweats. Avoiding spicy foods may help to limit night sweats. Also, keeping your bedroom at a comfortable and cool temperature, or using a fan or leaving a window open for fresh air may help. Taking a cool shower just before retiring to bed may also improve your situation. When night sweats do strike, try having a glass of ice water to cool your body down.

Heartburn Can Interfere With Healthy Sleep—What to Do

Sufferers of heartburn know what it is like to have difficulty sleeping. The painful condition seems to worsen at night, likely because of the reclined position. Gastroesophageal reflux disorder, or GERD, is commonly referred to as heartburn. Symptoms include a burning sensation in the chest. Other problems that can accompany heartburn include difficulty breathing, asthma symptoms, coughing and hoarse voice. The condition is caused by acid from the stomach backing up into the esophagus. Fortunately, this is a condition that is easily treated with a number of different medications.

Lifestyle changes and dietary adjustments can often lead to significant improvements in GERD symptoms. Avoiding things like chocolate, alcohol, fried foods, coffee or other foods with ingredients that may be difficult to digest or weaken the "seal" between the stomach and the esophagus may help.

Once inflammation occurs, avoiding anything that is acidic, such as citrus fruits, tomato based products, or spicy foods, can help to ease the discomfort associated with heartburn. Smoking can also make symptoms worse, so quitting is a great idea for helping heartburn—among other health benefits. Also, losing weight can provide some relief for many people suffering from heartburn.

Heartburn that worsens at night may be improved by adjusting the sleep position, particularly by raising the head of your bed by a few inches. This can be accomplished through certain commercially available products designed for this purpose, or simply propping the bed frame on some wooden blocks. Avoiding a completely reclined position, by doing this, can help to keep the stomach acid where it belongs—in the stomach. Also, avoiding eating for a few hours before going to bed can help, because the digestive process will be farther along.

There are a number of over the counter medications that are useful for treatment of heartburn, and your doctor may recommend that you try these for relief. Good old fashioned Rolaids, Tums and Maalox are often very helpful. If symptoms persist chronically, then seek medical attention to rule out more serious causes of heartburn.

More severe cases of heartburn may not be as responsive to the over the counter remedies and may require prescription medication to get relief. There are numerous prescription medications on the market today that give heartburn sufferers relief from the uncomfortable and painful burning sensation. Changing the amount of acid in the stomach will help to reduce the occurrence of heartburn   or   GERD.

For the most serious cases of heartburn, surgical intervention may be required. There is an operation, called a fundoplication, that improves the barrier between the stomach and the esophagus, helping to prevent acid from being pushed back in the wrong direction. Although the surgery is invasive and should be a "last resort," it can be very successful and there is a quick recovery.

Non-invasive procedures, such as the use of radio waves to treat gastroesophageal reflux disorder, are being investigated, with some success for many sufferers.

Neutralizing acid in the stomach by consuming bread products or bland foods can also help. Milk is known to be a natural stomach soother, and may help to absorb acid or minimize the effects. This may often help those who are experiencing heartburn when they are trying to go to sleep, but may only be a quick fix for the problem and other more significant treatments should be attempted as well.

Treatment of heartburn is often successful, and can help to improve your sleep if this is a problem for you. Heartburn while sleeping is especially painful and will cause major disruptions in the sleep cycle and your attempts at getting a good night's sleep. Making sure that you are addressing any underlying issues will be an important step in improving sleep patterns that are interrupted by heartburn symptoms.

Effects of Sleep Disorders on Learning and What to Do

Studies have shown that major learning problems are often associated with sleep disorders. More than 40 million people are affected in the United States alone by chronic sleep problems. With so many people working various shifts at their jobs, it can be difficult to establish healthy sleep hygiene routines and this can increase the number of people who suffer from sleep disorders. Those who have disrupted physical schedules or are very busy are at a higher risk for having significant sleep problems.

When left untreated, sleep problems can affect every aspect of a person's life, and the quality of life is significantly reduced. Add in the numerous health problems that are associated with sleep disorders and it becomes an epidemic problem.

Issues with learning, attention, concentration and behavior are more prevalent with people, especially children, with sleep disorders. Sleep deprivation is a serious problem and one that needs to be promptly and thoroughly addressed and treated before it causes even more problems. In adults, poor concentration can lead to injuries, distracted driving, poor job performance and mental health issues. Personal relationships are also affected by sleep problems.

Cognitive function decreases when sleep deprivation hits. Poor memory, slow reaction times and a limited ability to learn new information are all seen when a person does not get proper sleep. Our brains require a certain amount of rest in order to function properly.

Humans cannot survive without sleep, that is one thing that is certain. Brain regeneration happens when we rest, and the brain must regenerate regularly in order to continue to work effectively. The hippocampus is a part of the brain responsible for many parts of learning, memory and emotion, and it needs to be properly rested in order to accomplish those big tasks.

Sleep is essential for learning, and there have been many research studies to confirm this fact. Both adults and children are affected when learning is interrupted. Just because we are done with our formal academic training does not mean that learning ends. People must learn things on a regular basis to survive, and proper sleep is required in order for this to happen. Academic and job performance demand top brain functioning, and getting enough rest is critical for this to occur.

Memory is affected by poor sleep, so retaining information that has been learned is extremely difficult for those who have sleep disorders, chronic sleep deprivation or conditions that result in interruption of proper sleep patterns and poor sleep hygiene. Sleep plays such a significant role in our ability to perform all of the tasks of daily living, from learning to job performance, and there is a direct correlation between not getting enough sleep and having problems in any of these areas.

Those with problems related to sleep, those who are chronically fatigued and those who have health conditions that are interfering with healthy sleep should take action toward discovering the causes for the problems and getting proper treatment. When left untreated, sleep problems will lead to a myriad of life difficulties, yet treatments are available and can definitely help people be more productive and more effective in every aspect of their life.

Lifestyle changes, dietary changes, medications and other treatments can be used for treating sleep disorders, and if you are suffering from sleep problems—whatever they may be—you should leave no stone unturned when it comes to fixing the problem once and for all. Proper diet, exercise, and an overall healthy lifestyle may be all that it takes to fix your sleep problem, but if it does persist then there are definitely medical treatments that are known to be very effective and helpful.

Improved sleep will lead to an improved life, and this is usually the goal of most people. Keep your body and your brain healthy and functioning at top capacity by focusing on fixing sleep problems and getting a good night's rest, every night.

We Want Your Feedback on This Book!

Our main purpose is to make sure that our readers get value from the books we publish and that they have a good experience with all of our products. We are always working to improve our books and other products with every revision and update.

Every piece of feedback makes a difference in this process. And we would appreciate yours as well - whether it is good or bad.

Please take one minute to let us know what you thought by following this link:

http://checkmatemg.com/feedbacksleepdisorders/

www.ingramcontent.com/pod-product-compliance
Lightning Source LLC
Chambersburg PA
CBHW070839290526
45795CB00002B/912